Mindfulness for Beginners

Powerful Techniques to Be In the Moment and Live a Problem Free, Stress Free, Happy and Healthy Life

Contents

Chapter 1. What Mindfulness Really Is & What It Means

Mindfulness is actually a mindset that allows you to be constantly mindful of what you are doing, but when people commonly refer to mindfulness they are usually referring to mediation techniques that help you to live in the moment. Mindfulness mediation is a combination of techniques that helps to improve your general health mentally, emotionally, physically and even spiritually. It helps you to ground yourself, understand yourself, and balance out the negative energy in your life.

Why should you live with mindfulness in mind?

Many people go through life without understanding what they're doing or even why they're doing it. It is important that you understand this lifestyle technique so that you can live in the present. Most people live their entire lives focused on the future or fixated on the past. So many people never live in the present, which cuts down their enjoyment in life. It is easier to enjoy every moment, including the small things that happen in that moment to contribute to your happiness, if you are constantly being mindful.

What are some of the benefits of living like this?

There are many benefits to mindfulness and practicing the techniques that come with it, which you'll learn in this book. One of the main benefits is that it can help you reach a more stable state of being. If you are more stable, you're more likely to be calm. Staying calm is going to help you to process everything that is going on around you in the physical world as well as what is going on in your own head.

This will lead to gaining self-knowledge, boosting your immune system, reaching emotional stability and so much more. From sleeping to starting your day, there is a technique that can help you. From mindfulness of emotions to mindfulness of physical sensation, these techniques only take a few minutes, and the benefits far outweigh the time that you lose.

What is the best mindfulness technique to start with?

The best technique to master first is mindfulness of breathing, and that's because it is the best way to balance yourself with this method of meditation quickly and effectively. Of course, it is also the technique that is going to feed into all other techniques. Most of these techniques start with mindfulness of breathing because it is your go-to technique to center yourself and block out the external world.

To practice mindfulness of breathing, you need to start by sitting down somewhere where you won't be distracted. Next, make sure that you are comfortable and close your eyes. It is usually best if the room is dark. Your breathing is going to be your object of concentration, so start by breathing in through your nose slowly.

With mindfulness of breathing you won't be following the path of your breath all the way to your lungs, but instead you are going to make sure that you concentrate on what it feels to take a breath in through your nose. Concentrate on how it feels in your nostrils, how it feels for your chest to expand without following the breath. Then, take note of how it feels for that breath to leave your body through your mouth.

You're going to want to focus on your breathing alone, and some people can do this by counting if they're having trouble. It is usually recommended that you count your breathing on each exhale, and count all the way up to ten and then back down again until you get to one. This will note the end of your mindfulness of breathing exercise, and you will be able to open up your eyes. Some people keep their eyes closed for a moment longer, relishing in how relaxed your body should feel.

What does this have to do with your state of being?

During mindfulness of breathing, you are more likely to let go of stress and tension, which is why it is helpful for almost every benefit that you're trying to reap from these meditation methods and practices. Stress negatively affects you spiritually, emotionally, physically and even mentally. You need all of these aspects of yourself to be in order if you want to be the best you possible, and many of your goals and the stability you seek are within your reach.

All you have to do is practice one of these techniques at least once a day. Many people will practice more than once a day, but it's completely up to you. You may want to practice a technique more than once a day if you're trying to get multiple benefits from it or if you're trying to work on an issue that you may have, such as anger.

Does mindfulness come naturally?

For some people, these techniques come as naturally as breathing after their first session. However, you will find that for the majority of people the act of being mindful and using these techniques is something that is accomplished through discipline, practice and time. It is not something that will come naturally to you immediately, but the more you practice the easier it will become. It'll be hard to stay focused at first, and this is why it is important to learn tips and tricks along the way. Master mindfulness of breathing before you move forward, as it'll help you to move onto other techniques which may be harder or require more concentration.

Does mindfulness improve your life immediately?

You may be wondering if these techniques are going to drastically change your life immediately, and the answer is no. You will notice a difference in your mindset, and you'll naturally shift over time to becoming a more positive person. How much this process changes your life and how quickly depends on what you're trying to use it for and how often you're practicing any of these techniques.

If you are practicing throughout the day, at least once daily, you're more likely to notice results quickly, and you're more likely to notice a shift in your overall mental state and energy levels. Of course, if you're using more than one of these techniques, you're also going to notice a greater change because you're targeting your entire lifestyle instead of just small areas of it.

Chapter 2. Strengthen Your Immune System

Now that you know what this meditation technique really is, you're probably wondering how mindfulness can help you. It can actually help your physical health, and this is because mindfulness can truly help your immune system. If you have a bad immune system, it's important that you add mindfulness and everything it has to offer to your daily regime. Of course, it's helpful even if you have a decent immune system to start with as well.

How does mindfulness help with your immune system?

As you'll learn these techniques are a meditation form that will help you to reduce your stress, and in turn this is going to make sure that your immune system is up and roaring to go. It doesn't matter what particular technique you're going to use. What matters is that you use one, and doing so on a regular basis is what will help you to reap the benefit of this form of meditation.

Is there another reason that mindfulness helps your immune system?

Yes, there is another reason that this practice is believed to help your immune system, and that's because as you turn your mind inward you become more in tune with your body mentally and physically. This allows your mind to be more aware of any illness you may be feeing, even on a subconscious level.

Many people believe that this is one reason that the immune system may pick up, helping us to

fight off any illness as it comes. You're more
likely to notice small symptoms of illness when
you are practicing mindful meditation because
you'll notice your body as a whole. You'll be
able to tell if your throat is slightly sore, if your
muscle aches, if you're feeling hotter than usual
and so on.

Your mental state is also known to affect your
immune system. If you are more positive, your
immune system is higher because there is less
holding it down. If you are experiencing
emotional trauma, even subconsciously, you
will lower your immune system because the
effects of anxiety will sink in, which can also
lead to depression.

Mindfulness meditation, just like meditation as
a whole, is known to help produce more
antibodies and stimulate immune system
regions of the brain. This helps to stimulate

your immune system as a whole. However, the effects aren't immediate, and sometimes a noticeable effect will take up to eight weeks.

What are the benefits of a raised immune system?

If you have a raised immune system it's going to keep your stress levels down, and they're down in the first place to help your immune system. This means that you're more likely to be a more positive person. You're also more likely to be able to handle the disappointments that come to you without falling into depression or experiencing too much anxiety about small issues. With a raised immune system one of the most obvious and beneficial benefits is that you won't be as likely to get sick.

This is useful all year round, but you'll also find that it's extremely useful during flu and cold season. If you get sick, you're more likely to fall into a rut, feel depression, miss work, lack concentration, and feel generally frazzled, making your quality of life go down. It can be hard to recover from being sick both physically and mentally, but with this form of meditation creating a boosted immune system, you're much more likely to be able to avoid the entire process.

Does it matter what mindfulness meditation that you use?

No it doesn't matter what type of meditation technique you use. All forms of this meditation are meant to center you, and this is what will help you to boost your immune system. Of course, mindfulness of breathing is one of the easiest exercises to work into your daily routine. Just make sure that you have at least ten minutes dedicated to these exercises.

There are different varieties of these practices that can be implemented to reach the benefit of a raised immune system, and it doesn't even matter where you practice. You can practice on the bus, at home, and even in nature. Adding nature into your mindfulness meditation practice will help as well, since nature is also known to help boost the immune system as well as improving your general attitude.

Does it have to be done in a routine to achieve this benefit?

Yes, to achieve this benefit you do need to make a routine of it. It is best to practice one of these techniques at least once daily for any benefit that it has to offer. However, you'll find that if you're trying to boost your immune system all you need to do is practice at least once daily for ten to fifteen minutes. You can improve your chances of boosting your immune system drastically by practicing in nature, in a quiet place, or more than once daily. Just remember that the effects of a boosted immune system do not show immediately, and just because you are unsure if it is working doesn't mean you should stop your practices. Instead, keep it up, as it may take up to eight weeks to notice an effect.

Chapter 3. Reach Emotional Stability

Your emotional stability will actually feed into a lot of different aspects of your life no matter if it's spiritual, physical, or mental. It's important that you have emotional stability, but it's actually hard for many people to reach a level of emotional stability that allows them to handle almost any situation in a healthy manner. Mindfulness can help you to reach emotional stability as well, and it's an easy benefit to reach.

So how does mindfulness help emotional stability directly?

There are many reasons that these techniques will help you to achieve emotional stability, and once again one of the reasons is that it'll help you to reduce the stress in your life. It also gives you a routine that you can follow, and during these meditations and practices, you work on grounding and centering yourself. This will allow you to observe your emotions.

By recognizing your emotions without trying to deny them, you are more easily able to accept your emotions. Every emotion should be accepted, no matter if it's justifiable or not. You cannot stop feeling certain emotions if you want to be emotionally stable, but instead you need to make sure that you can just filter out your negative emotions, accept them, and change your perspective to something a little more positive.

What are the benefits of having a stable emotional state?

There are many benefits to stabilizing your emotions, and one of the biggest benefits is that you won't have to deal with negativity hanging over you. When you have a stable emotional state, you're much more likely to view the world in a positive manner. You'll be able to filter out negative emotions, and you'll be able to handle difficult situations with a little more ease.

It'll even help you in times of anger, and it'll help you to forgive people. You may not want to forgive people, but keep in mind that when you have a forgiving nature you're more likely to have less stress. This is because when you're holding a grudge you're spending time and energy on people who don't deserve it, but you're free from that when you forgive someone.

Is there a mindfulness meditation that is best for your emotional state?

Yes, there actually is. You'll want to practice mindfulness of emotions if you want to get the best results when centering yourself and stabilizing your emotional state. Emotional stability has many benefits, but it can be hard to achieve without proper guidance. Mindfulness of emotion is a great way to guide you through your emotions, learning to work on one at a time.

From acceptance to changing your perspective on your emotions, mindfulness of emotions can help you with it all. Over time when you practice it regularly, the practice becomes almost second nature. This is the increased stability of your emotional state, and it means that it'll be both easier to manage and upkeep.

How do you practice mindfulness of emotions?

Like all of these meditation forms you need to start by relaxing and getting comfortable. Make sure that there is no tension in your shoulders, so make sure to be in a comfortable position and then close your eyes. You'll need to focus internally, so don't let the external world distract you. Try to be in a quiet environment, and start with basic breathing exercises. Count your breaths one to ten. Make sure to breathe in through your nose and out through your mouth, paying attention to how it feels for that breath to go from your nostrils to your lungs and back out again.

Once your attention is finally focused you can then turn your attention to any strong emotion that you're feeling at the time. This can be anything from anger to anxiety to happiness. You can use both positive and negative emotions. Pick an emotion you're either feeling or a strong one you can pull up. Pull up the memory of what caused that emotion so that you can truly connect with, letting it wash over you.

Keep your eyes closed and your focus on that emotion, trying to recall everything that led up to it, including any senses you may remember. Imagine the situation, walking yourself through it all over again. You'll feel a sensation in your body, and let thought enter your mind. Do not entertain the thoughts, and instead just let them float by, only acknowledging them. Ask yourself what emotion you're feeling and if there is more than one.

Try to look at the event in a curious manner, looking to see what caused everything to happen. This will help you to keep from denying the emotion. Recognize any physical sensation that is happening as well, such as if your heart is pounding or your muscles are tensing up. This will help you to become more aware, but never judge the emotion. Remember that you shouldn't feel guilty or stressed over this emotion. Tell yourself it's natural, and when you feel you have accepted the emotion you'll want to go back to concentrating on breathing. Then you can open your eyes.

Will you see effects from practicing mindfulness of emotion right away?

Yes, you'll start to feel more stable. However, you won't reach full emotional stability for a while. You'll need to keep practicing, at least once daily, to make sure that there is no buildup of negative emotions. Negative emotions decrease the stability of your emotional state, which will in turn lead to depression, stress, anxiety and bouts of rage or anger.

When is the best time to practice this type of meditation to help?

You can practice mindfulness of emotion anytime if you want to cultivate a stable emotional state. Of course, you'll also want to make sure you practice it on a regular basis, and doing so at least once a day is recommended. If you feel a particularly strong emotion, then you can choose to accept that emotion and learn from it so long as you accept the emotion. Mindfulness of emotion is meant to help you accept these emotions and balance your emotional state overall.

Chapter 4. Help Yourself in Moments of Anger

Anger is something that affects everyone from time to time, and you need to know how to handle it properly if you want to live a healthy life. Anger affects our overall mood, and it can lead to unneeded stress and anxiety. Of course, these techniques can help with your moments of anger as well. It can help you to walk away from a frustrating and anger producing situation, but it can also help you reach a type of stability in your inner self that will help you to be less likely to be angered as easily in the first place.

Isn't anger natural and shouldn't it be accepted?

Yes, anger is natural, and it does need to be accepted. However, there is a difference between accepting your anger and acting on your anger. When you are in the moment, you're more likely to act on your anger than accepting it. Anger has many negative effects on your life, and you should make sure that you try and balance out these negative effects.

Anger can affect your family as well, as it makes you feel worse, which makes you more likely to lash out at others. If you are feeling down or negative, that will affect those around you as well. You need to feel more positive if you want positivity in your life. Anger can even affect your health, such as your heart health. It can raise your risk of stroke, heart attack, and high blood pressure. It's best to stay away from anger whenever possible, and you should never dwell on anger. It can help with both limiting your anger as well as accepting it so that you can move forward with your life.

How does this technique help you in moments of anger?

This can be a tricky question because it's hard to handle anger when you're in the moment. However, it does a good job at guiding you along the way. The act of being mindful is to be aware of your mental, physical, emotional and spiritual state. Your entire being will go out of balance when you're angry, and these techniques, including meditation, are meant to help put you back into balance.

This is no different when dealing with anger, but the process is a little harder to handle. Practicing this technique before you try to use it to help your anger is best because it will help you to understand the process and go into the needed state of mind even during anger, when you're in a state of emotional distress.

What is one exercise you can practice immediately if you start to get angry?

You'll want to make yourself aware of the anger that you're feeling, and you need to turn inward to see what physical sensation is going through you. Make your mind aware of what your body is going through because during anger it is too likely that you'll separate your body and mind to help you cope with the rage that you're feeling. You may notice sensations in your face, chest, or even your stomach. Your heart rate or breathing may increase, and your muscles are likely to tense up. Make sure to observe any and all reactions in your body.

Next, you need to remind yourself to breathe, just like you would during mindfulness of breathing. Breathe in and imagine that breath going to where you're feeling these physical sensations, cleansing the area. You can close your eyes if it makes it easier, and for many people it will. Start to count each breath you take, and keep counting until you get to ten. Imagine that every time you breathe out a little more of that anger is released from your body.

Keep with the sensation of breathing as well as the sensations that you are feeling from anger. Observe these sensations as they increase or lessen, and learn to accept it.

Next, you'll start to turn more inward, allowing yourself to actually notice your thoughts. You may think your situation isn't fair, that you have a right to be mad, and that you won't take anymore. Any and all thoughts you have don't need to be justified. You just need to accept these thoughts. Let them pass through your mind, but try not interact on these thoughts or you'll end up dwelling on them and the anger that they're causing.

This will help you to dissipate the majority of your anger. Once you feel your anger lessen, you'll be able to see exactly what you're doing in the situation, even if it's not yet clear what you should do next. With most of the anger out of your system, you can then look for a solution and communicate a little better. Remember to stay honest and cope with your anger whenever it occurs.

Does this need to be done on a regular basis?

You can practice any of these techniques on a regular basis, but that doesn't mean you have to practice the technique above every single day. It will help if you practice mindfulness of emotion every day because it will help you to learn to accept your emotions, including anger, a little easier. This will help you to control anger as it rises up in the moment as well as deal with the after effects of anger much easier.

You will want to make the above practice a practice for every time you feel angry. You'll find that it is much easier to let anger go, and it'll even be easier to understand why you're angry and solve the problem. If you don't know why you're angry or how to solve a problem, that is only going to compound your anger and make the situation that much worse.

Chapter 5. Strengthen Personal Relationships

One of the biggest issues in any relationship is the conflicts that you're bound to get into. Of course, there can be multiple reasons that your personal relationships are suffering, and there are many different types of personal relationships. You have to be in a good place mentally, emotionally and physically if you want to be able to hold your own in any personal relationship, and this practice is known to help with this. It will help you to balance yourself, helping you to gain a more positive outlook and increase positive interactions.

How can it help you with your personal relationships?

You'll find that this practice will help you with any of your personal relationships for a multitude of reasons, but one of the main reasons is that it will help you to understand yourself a little better. The more time you spend during these meditation practices, the more you'll be able to learn about yourself. This is how you gain self-knowledge, which will be covered more in depth in a later chapter. When you understand a little more about yourself, such as faults, strengths and even issues that you may not yet have resolved, you'll be able to make sure you aren't taking out your problems on other people.

It is important in a healthy relationship that you handle each problem that you have, between you and the other person or just any personal problems, in a mature and effective manner. You can't do this unless you're able to identify the problem, which the self-knowledge that it can provide will help with. Understanding these techniques will also help you to let go of any grudges, and this is because mindfulness can help you to let go of both the anger that is causing any of your issues with someone else as well as see the issue more clearly.

If you are wrapped up in the event with the thoughts and emotions that the event caused swirling around you, you're much less likely to see the event clearly. You may even be at fault or at least partially at fault, but with clouded vision you'll never know. It is known to help you achieve this clarity by allowing you to experience and recognize your thoughts and emotions without having to immerse yourself in them.

Thoughts and emotions always have to play their course, but if you fuel them then it'll just cause more gasoline to be put on a fire that will only get harder to put out. It is healthier to see situations of frustration, anger, or just tense situations more clearly when you're in a relationship because it'll help to make sure you don't cast undue blame or act out unfairly. When you're more reasonable, the relationship is more likely to last and stay healthy.

Will this practice help you to forgive the people in your life?

Yes, it is able to help you forgive people as well. One of the ways that it helps with forgiveness is that it helps you to understand that things happen, and once you view the situation clearly you may be able to understand why people acted the way they did. You're also more likely to see the role that you've played in events as well.

You can even use this practice to forgive someone by altering mindfulness of emotion. If you need to forgive somewhere, there is always a reason and usually it's related to anger or some other negative emotion. Make sure to draw that emotion up when you're practicing mindfulness of emotion. Make sure that you observe the event that makes you need to forgive that person, but when you're concentrating on the details you need to concentrate on that person.

Let everything but that person and the anger you feel towards them fade from your mind. Your thoughts will still play out about them, but observe them without interacting. Observe the emotions looking at that person's face causes you, but don't fuel those emotions or interact with them. Next, you're going to want to speak this part in your head, but you can also speak it out loud if you think it'll work best.

Tell yourself that you forgive that person. Tell them that they can no longer hurt you. That you'll let the anger go. You may have to repeat it a few times if you want to truly let it take effect. Now, concentrate on your breathing as you turn that mantra inwards. Make sure that you concentrate on any residual anger that you are feeling towards them while you're breathing in and out.

With each breath, imagine that anger leaving your body, keeping your eyes closed. Concentrate on how the breath travels from your nostrils to your lungs, expanding your chest and leaving your lungs, removing your breath and anger from your body through your mouth. Keep this up until you truly feel like you forgive the person, and then you can open your eyes.

How else does mindfulness help with personal relationships?

It will help with your personal relationships because it will help to ground and balance you. With these techniques being practiced on a daily basis, you'll feel more stable and more positive. These techniques are meant to help balance your spiritual, mental, emotional and physical state.

It'll help you to boost your immune system, relieve stress, and even get rid of negative energy. If you are more positive and healthy, you are more likely to react in a healthy manner to everything that is going on around you. That positivity will also spread to everything that is around you, including your personal relationships. This allows for those relationships to grow and flourish.

How do you reap this benefit from practicing mindfulness?

Remember that it comes with routine, and it'll be gained over time. You won't see an immediate improvement in how you react with everyone around you. You won't see it making your love life better immediately, but you will see an increase in positivity immediately as these meditation techniques are practiced. Just be patient, and you'll be able to reap this benefit over time.

Chapter 6. Gain Self-Awareness & Understanding

Most people do not really know themselves, who they are, or what really makes themselves tick. This is what self-knowledge is supposed to help you gain, and there are many benefits to gaining self-knowledge. You are better able to understand your own actions and reactions, even involuntary ones, if you can truly understand yourself. It is able to help you understand yourself, but it's not a quick process to do so. There is always something new that you can learn about who you are and why you act the way you do.

Why do you need to gain self-knowledge?

Self-knowledge is something that most people don't have, but there are many benefits to gaining it, such as being able to understand your own emotions. Many people just feel emotions without understanding them, and yes mindfulness of emotions can help you. However, mindfulness of emotion is more so meant to help you understand how to accept and move past emotions. It will not be enough to help you fully understand why you are experiencing certain emotions. There are many times that people are confused by themselves.

If you understand yourself, you are much less likely to be frustrated in certain situations, and this will help you to process things quicker, easier, and in a healthier manner. You're much less likely to rely on vices like alcohol, denial, or even drugs. Instead, you'll be able to move past things in a healthy manner as they come up, and it improves coping mechanisms as well.

You'll also be able to understand why certain patterns in your life keep happening, bringing you clarity. You need clarity to understand how to break out of a rut you may be in, but you need clarity of self which these techniques can provide when practiced properly.

What is the best practice for gaining self-knowledge?

Almost any one of these techniques when practiced will help you to gain self-knowledge, but mindfulness of thought is practiced most commonly for this benefit. If you're looking to start a mindfulness of thought session, you should know that it may take a little longer than other techniques. This is because you have to account for the time it takes to observe many thoughts so that you can take in the process and ideas into yourself to process later. A mindfulness of thought session may last twenty minutes or more. Some people do have sessions that are ten minutes long, but at least fifteen minutes is usually best.

Just like any other one of these exercises, you are going to want to start in a comfortable position with little to no outside distractions around you, so that you can turn internally. Start with mindfulness of breathing, and when you feel comfortable that you have blocked out the external world, you can move onto turning your consciousness inward instead of on the physical sensation of breathing.

Observe what's bothering you or what you're thinking of. You may just be thinking that it's peaceful, and that's fine as well. Do not interact with the thought, as this can be detrimental to the process. You do not want to change the way you think or you won't be able to observe yourself properly. Allow your thoughts to wander, and there is no reason to reign them or put them in a certain direction.

No matter what comes up, try to stay disconnected from your thoughts. Do not exasperate your thoughts, and do not comment on your thoughts. It is not meant to be a conversation with yourself. Try not to judge your own thoughts. It doesn't matter if your thoughts are cruel or even sad. You need to just let them flow freely. You can later reflect on what you've learned about yourself, but you should not do that while you are just trying to observe.

Once you feel like you've observed your thoughts for long enough because you feel your mind trying to push your thoughts in a particular direction, you'll need to end the session. Return to a mindfulness of breathing exercise before opening your eyes. Many people find it best to sit there for a moment, and others find that it is useful to write down what they'd want to reflect on because there is so much going through their mind. Other people find that their mind is still relatively calm, but it is usually important to write down anything that you want to further experience or understand.

How does this help you gain self-knowledge?

What you've learned from yourself will help you to handle everything that is thrown your way. You're going to want to make sure that you reflect on everything if you want to gain the self-knowledge you seek. You may not truly understand how your own brain works, but by observing your thoughts you see patterns in your thinking, and it can help you see cause and effect of what's happening in your life and in your mental and emotional state. Once you recognize these patterns you'll be able to change them or at least accept them, which can help you to change your coping mechanisms as well. This can help you to improve your overall life.

Is there a best time of day to practice mindfulness of thought?

No there is no particular time of day that you have to practice mindfulness of thoughts to reap the benefits that it has to offer. However, many people find that it's easier to practice mindfulness of thought right before bed or right after they get up in the morning. If you choose to practice mindfulness of thought in the morning before you start your day, you're more likely to feel centered and grounded during the day. This will also have a positive impact on your life and how you interact with the world around you, including the people in it.

Chapter 7. Boost Overall Concentration

It can also help to boost your overall concentration, and this can help you in many facets of your life. Concentration will help you to succeed in many different ways, including business and school. If you have increased concentration, you are more likely to make sure that you accomplish anything you put your mind too. This is because you'll be able to put more of your mind into everything you're doing, and you're much less likely to become distracted by simple things.

You don't need to have ADD or ADHD to become distracted, but even if you do, it can actually help with that as well. It's just a little harder, and it might take a little longer to see some results if you suffer from an actual disorder. Everyone can use a concentration boost, and with these practices that boost can come easy.

How does increased concentration help you to reach success?

When your focus and concentration is increased, as stated above, you're much more likely to succeed in anything that you try to do. When you're trying to learn a new hobby, for example, you'll find that it takes concentration to gain the knowledge needed. It also takes concentration to practice many hobbies, such as wood working, leather working, jewelry making, writing or even embroidery. It doesn't matter what your hobby is, but if you can focus yourself it'll turn out better.

You'll also find that you'll be able to reach personal goals that you set if you can concentrate on your daily activities. This is because procrastination lessens, helping you to accomplish more, which will in turn give you more free time. More free time will help you to increase your positivity, which is something that these techniques help with in the first place.

For example, if you're reading, you'll find that concentration will help you to read a little faster. If you're trying, you'll find that if you focus on what you're typing, you're probably going to type faster as well. This will help you to get your work done faster, and it'll help you to gain the knowledge for your work or just about anything faster.

You'll still have the ability to multi-task, and concentration will actually help with that as well. If you can concentrate on one particular activity, you're more likely to be able to concentrate on a variety of activities because your mind is trained towards focusing.

What mindfulness method is best when you're trying to increase concentration?

There isn't any particular method that will help you with concentration more than others. Instead, you'll find that just about any one of these techniques will help you to concentrate naturally. You'll learn how to block out the external world, and this means that you'll even be able to block out the external world expect for what you're working on. This is demonstrated when you're using mindfulness of breathing, for example, and that's because you're concentrating on the physical sensation of breathing.

Concentrating on physical sensation is one way to immerse yourself in anything that you're doing. Take typing for example, if you can immerse your mind in the feeling of typing, then you're more likely to keep typing without distraction. You'll be able to observe the thoughts that come to mind as you write, but you won't have to interact with them. Instead, you'll just transcribe the thoughts that are relevant by typing them, helping you to succeed in what you were trying to type up.

Are there any other ways that mindfulness will help you to concentrate better?

Yes, it will help you to concentrate by removing internal stresses naturally as well. When you're not settled mentally or emotionally, then you won't be able to concentrate on anything that you're doing physically. Your mind won't even be able to hold a thought most of the time, no less acting on something that will lead to success.

Instead, you need to calm down your mental and emotional state so that you can reach a stable point which will allow you to work. Often, it will help you to do this naturally, but there are times that you can use a technique to accomplish this immediately even if you are not naturally settled. Just take a technique, whichever one you feel is most applicable, and use it to calm your mental state and balance out your energies.

If you really feel too unbalanced, going and practicing any one of these meditation methods in nature can help. Nature is naturally calming, and it can act as a stress relief. Remember that stress can actually block concentration, just like anxiety and depression. This is why you should never let your emotional state build up until it's out of control. Handle everything as it comes, and you'll find that your mindfulness sessions can be shorter even though they're a little more frequent.

This makes them that much more effective, helping you to reap the benefits of everything that this practice has to offer. You can concentrate on mindfulness of breathing if you want to clear your thoughts, or you can use mindfulness of emotion if something specific is bothering you, but mindfulness of physical sensation can help as well which is where you take stock of everything that is affecting your body, including the tension and aches that you feel.

Does it help if you practice this technique regularly?

Just like if you're practicing mindfulness regularly for any other benefit that it has to offer, you'll find that practicing it regularly will also help you with concentration. It'll become easier and easier to concentrate the more you practice, as your mind is a muscle that you can exercise. Concentration is one of those things that takes practice, and your focus can actually sharpen over time. This is why it can help you find a permanent solution to concentration and focus problems, even if you're suffering from a medical condition like ADD or ADHD. Just remember that it may take weeks to notice a difference, but some people will notice a difference in days.

Chapter 8. Reach Your Weight Loss Goals

Everyone has a few weight loss goals every once in a while. Some people want to lose more weight than others, and that's fine. No matter how much or how little weight you want to lose, you'll want to use it to help reach your weight loss goals. There are many different techniques that you can use to help you reach every weight loss goal you had in the time that you wanted to.

How does mindfulness help with your weight loss goals?

It is known to reduce stress, which will help you to lose weight. When you are less stressed, you're less likely to be anxious or depressed. Anxiousness or depression can also lead to weight gain, but even if you already anxious or depressed, these techniques will help with that. You need to center yourself, and then you'll be able to help improve your overall mood and energy levels. When you're more positive, you have more energy in the first place.

How much weight can mindfulness help you lose?

It can help you reach all of your weight loss goals, and it's great in helping you to maintain the weight you want as well. Basic techniques can help you maintain your weight because it reduces your stress. Stress has been proven to worsen weight gain as well as self-control, which will lead to mindless eating that will also make you put weight on. There will be a point that weight loss will lessen and seem to come a plateau when you're using any of these techniques to help you lose weight, but if you're patient you'll be able to push past it to lose more weight so long as you're practicing it with a healthy lifestyle as well.

What mindfulness practice is best to help you lose weight?

Mindfulness of eating practices are the best to help you lose weight. Many people aren't aware of just how much they're eating, and many people will sit down and eat a bag of chips without realizing exactly what they've done and how many calories they've consumed. This is one of the main reasons that people tend to gain weight. Mindfulness of eating will help you to enjoy your food while you are still making sure that everything you eat is portion controlled, even the bad foods.

Mindfulness of eating is the act of eating with your five senses. Take a small bite of food and take it with you, sitting down comfortably. Next, you're going to want to turn off any distractions. Make sure that you tune out the external world, and mindfulness of breathing is usually the best way to center yourself so that you're not distracted. Then start by smelling your food. Enjoy the scent of what the food smells like. Concentrate on what the food feels like in your fingers or when placed to your lips. Look at the food, and take note of how appetizing the food looks to you. If there's any sound, try to appreciate that sound like if a bag is crinkling, and then once you've appreciated the food, take a small bite of it.

No matter how small the food piece is, try to make it at least two bites. Savor the food, chewing slowly. Eat only a few bites at a time, and you should feel more satisfied than if you were eating mindlessly. Concentrate on how the taste lingers on your tongue as you transitioning yourself back to breathing, and then open your eyes to go back about your day. If you practice mindfulness of eating, you're much less likely to mindlessly eat to gain weight as well as enjoy your food a little more.

So do you need to use a proper diet and exercise, or is mindfulness enough?

It is a great way to get a head start on your weight loss goals, but it's not enough to help you lose all of the weight you want. You may lose a few pounds with this technique on its own, but you'll never lose a lot without the proper diet and exercise. Remember that exercise will help to boost your metabolism, making all of your weight loss efforts that much more effective. Burn off the calories you eat, even when you are using mindfulness of eating practices. A proper diet is also necessary because you won't lose weight if you're eating foods that are bad for you, and even if you do by cutting back on the amount you consume, it won't be sustainable weight loss on its own.

Will you see results quickly or does it take a while when trying to lose weight with mindfulness?

Sadly, actual weight loss will take time, just like any other method of weight loss. However, you should notice that you feel much more satisfied after you use mindfulness of eating, and you're more likely to appreciate your food a little more as well. This will mean that you won't have to eat as much to feel as satisfied. You'll even notice when you're full a little easier, which will help you to stop eating when you're full instead of continuing to eat because you're not giving yourself time to fully feel the effects of the food on your stomach.

If you eat too quickly, it's proven that you're much likely to eat too much. You can practice mindfulness of eating anytime you want to, and some people even practice a version during every meal. Just make sure that you aren't eating with distraction because it will pull you out of your exercise and negate the positive effects that you'd get from it.

This is why eating in a room by yourself or at least at a table without any distractions, such as TV or the computer, is usually recommended when you're trying to lose weight. It doesn't matter if you exercise before mindfulness of eating, but many people still prefer exercising afterwards so they can burn off the calories. The positivity will also tend to give you more energy for your exercise routine.

Chapter 9. Help Your Sleep & Dreams

Everyone knows that sleep is extremely important, and dreams are important as well. You'll feel more positive when you have enough sleep and you've had positive dreams. Luckily, if you are more positive overall, positive dreams will come naturally as well. Experiencing your dream cycle will help you to feel more rested at night so long as they are positive dreams, and the amount of sleep you get will affect every facet of your life. If you're too tired, you're much more likely to do poorly in work, school or even at social events. Negativity can hang on your energy if you aren't getting enough sleep, and not sleeping can lead to a variety of medical problems as well.

What is the importance of sleeping and dreaming?

As stated above, one of the main benefits of getting enough sleep and dreaming during it is that you'll be able to act more positively and view the world in a more positive manner. Better sleep will also help to ease chronic pain, improve heart health, and help to deter serious health issues like heart attacks, obesity and diabetes. If you're getting enough sleep, you're also less likely to become injured, and this is because sleep deprivation can cause many disasters, including car accidents.

It'll increase your general mood and positivity, which will help you to be more productive and reach whatever goals that you put out, and it'll help you to keep your weight under control. Sleep and good dreams lowers your stress, which is also needed for positive interactions.

You're also able to make better decisions when you have sleep because you have a clearer head, and you're known for being less irrational. Not to mention that it can improve your immune system as well as your memory.

How does it help your sleep and your dreams?

You may be wondering how this meditation form will help you to dream better and improve sleep as a whole, and one of the main ways is that it removes anything that is stressing you out to the point that you can't sleep. With these practices, you'll learn how to remove these stress factors internally, and it can even help your aches and pains. For example, one of the main reasons that people have trouble sleeping is that a problem they are facing is stressing them out.

It is also known to help you with clarity, and you'll want to try mindfulness of breathing to help relax you as well. The clarity you gain from these practices will help you to put your problems into perspective. Of course, you'll also find that there is progressive muscle relaxation that you can use when you are using these techniques, and that will help you to get to sleep as well, as aches and pains can keep you up.

If you're feeling angry at a particular person, you can also use mindfulness of emotions to help. The version of mindfulness that helps with forgiveness is also best if you're trying to make yourself forgive someone so that they stop affecting your sleep and dreams. If you're having too many nightmares, mindfulness of breathing before bed for anxiety reasons is usually recommended.

What is the best exercise to help you with sleep?

As stated above, mindfulness of breathing and mindfulness of emotions is going to help you get to sleep as well. However, you'll find that mindfulness of physical sensation is extremely helpful when you are trying to get to sleep. You'll need at least fifteen minutes to do it, but the process is actually pretty easy. Just start by closing your eyes after you've found a comfortable position to sit or lay down in.

Focus all of your attention on mindfulness of breathing at first, and experience the breathing. You should feel yourself riding each of your breaths as if you were riding waves, and pay attention to how it moves through your body. Afterwards, you'll want to shift your awareness to the feel of sitting. Pay close attention to how it feels to sit against the chair. Notice all of the parts that are in contact with the chair. Try to immerse yourself in that feeling, and allow yourself to just exist in that moment.

Next, start to take stock of your body, and allow yourself to expand your awareness to your body as a whole. Recognize if there is a breeze against your arms, if you feel cold, or even if there are any aches or pains in your body. Notice if you're experiencing thirst or hunger. Make sure to take stock of all of the physical sensations that you're feeling.

Remember that you should never judge any experience, just like you wouldn't judge any emotion. You also don't want to label any sensation because this will snap you out of your physical awareness, and you shouldn't hunt for a sensation. Don't ask yourself if you are hungry, but instead just take note of it if you notice it when you expand your consciousness.

Allow yourself to feel all of that, and once you feel you've fully immersed yourself into physical sensation for a little while, try and shift your attention back to how it feels for your body to make contact with the chair. Then, shift it to how it feels to breath. Allow yourself to feel that once more for a few moments before you open your eyes.

Is there a best time to practice mindfulness of physical sensation to improve your sleep and dreams?

Yes, the best time to practice mindfulness of physical sensation is right before you go to bed. This will help you to relax right before bed, and it'll help you to release any tension that you may be having. This should allow you to drift off to sleep without anything bothering your mind, consciously or subconsciously. Of course, other exercises can also be performed throughout the day and right before bed to help you with better sleep and dreams as well.

Chapter 10. Always Keep These Tips & Tricks in Mind

There are still tips and tricks to mindfulness that you can apply if you're having trouble, as it'll help to ease you into the process as well as help you to just understand mindfulness as a whole. Once you've mastered mindfulness of breathing, everything else should come a little more naturally, but that doesn't quite make it natural.

Avoid Jewelry:

It may seem strange at first, but it is usually best that you avoid jewelry if you're trying to practice any of these mindful techniques. This is because jewelry is distracting. It is shiny if you have your eyes open, heavy, jingles, and it can sometimes pinch. This is more likely to make you aware and keep you aware of the physical world around you when you are trying to pull your thoughts somewhere else so that you can practice a technique. You can just temporarily remove this jewelry, but it's better if the distraction isn't there when you get started.

Avoid Uncomfortable Clothing:

Uncomfortable clothing should be avoided for the same reason that you'd want to avoid jewelry when you're trying to practice any of these techniques. This is because any of these practices and techniques require concentration on a specific aspect of what you are feeling, experiencing, or doing. You do not want to be distracted by something that is pinching you, too tight, or making you feel suffocated. Yoga pants are actually recommended, but anything you feel comfortable in will do. Remove things like belts or uncomfortable shoes before starting any exercise or technique.

Practice One Technique at a Time:

Don't try to move onto other mindfulness techniques unless you have really mastered mindfulness of breathing. Mindfulness of breathing is like your foundation that will help you build up your knowledge of mindfulness, helping you to practice it properly. You can then move onto another technique, but never try to really learn more than one at a time. Eventually, you should know every technique that you want to, but you'll find out that it does take time if you don't want to overwhelm yourself.

Try to Avoid Light:

Unless a mindfulness technique requires you to see something, it is usually best to practice in a dark room. This is because even when your eyes are closed, you'll see a red tinge to your eyelids as the light tries to filter through. It is easier for you to concentrate internally if you're not being distracted by lighting. Of course, black out curtains are recommended.

You can practice this meditation form in sunlight, especially if you want to practice outside, but it's not recommended if you're a beginner. If you want to practice outside, try to practice in the shade where the lighting that you're seeing from behind your eyes is less likely to change due to cloud coverage or other shadows flickering through the light that's being cast on you.

Remember Not to Judge:

Part of being mindful is to live in the moment without judging the moment, and that can be very hard to master. It is within human nature to judge and label things, including ourselves and what we feel and experience. If you are truly experiencing the present, you are not allowing yourself to tint the experience with your judgements. This is why you should try not to judge what you're feeling, especially if you are practicing mindfulness of thoughts or emotion. Judging can ruin the entire thing. You can later reflect on your experience, and this is the time that will allow you to label anything that you want, but you should still try to avoid labeling anything negatively.

Get Rid of Negativity as It Comes:

It is harder to be mindful and positive if you let negativity build within you or around you. This is why part of being mindful successfully is doing so regularly. If you are experiencing negativity in your emotions, feeling down for some unknown reason, having issues sleeping, experiencing nightmares or anything else that is causing negativity, then practice mindfulness so that you can let it go. Letting it go is important, as it helps you to rebalance yourself, which improves your positivity and reduces stress in your overall life.

Don't Become Frustrated:

You need to try and not become frustrated, even if you're having a hard time being mindful. This is because this is a mediation practice that is hard for many people, and you can't expect to be a natural at it. Experiencing true mindfulness will require patience and practice, so you have to have the time to dedicate to it. You won't see immediate benefits, at least not drastic ones, but you will experience these benefits if you practice these methods diligently and successfully. However, if you become frustrated you are allowing negativity and stress to enter your being and your life. This will block you from being mindful successfully. So stick to it, and be patient.

Make a Routine:

It is important that you try and make a routine out of any one of these practices. This will help you buckle down and practice like you need to so that you'll become successful. It is usually best to practice mindfulness at least once a day, and if you set a time aside for it in the first place, you're more likely to stick with it. This will allow you to develop the diligence that you need to decrease your stress and open yourself up to the benefits that are amiable to you.

There is no time of day that you have to practice mindfulness, but try doing so at least in the morning or at night. These are the two most successful times to practice mindfulness without interruption. Just make sure that you're awake enough if you choose to do it in the morning, since it is meant to help relax you enough so that you can start your day on a positive foot. Sadly, this means that you do run the risk of falling asleep. This is why many people will choose to practice it at night, especially if they are having issues sleeping.